THE

ESSENTIAL

GUIDE TO

CHAIR YOGA

FOR SENIORS

SCIENCE-BACKED EXERCISES TO
IMPROVE YOUR STRENGTH, MOBILITY,
BALANCE, AND RECLAIM YOUR
INDEPENDENCE

CONTENTS

1

WELCOME NOTE FROM THE AUTHOR

D ear Reader,

Welcome to "The Essential Guide to Chair Yoga for Seniors." I am Laura Garrett, your guide and companion on this transformative journey towards a healthier, more balanced, and fulfilling life. As we embark on this path together, I want to share not only the practices and knowledge I've accumulated over the years but also the warmth, encouragement, and understanding that have been the cornerstone of my teaching.

You might be wondering, why chair yoga? Perhaps you're at a stage in life where the traditional forms of exercise seem daunting, or maybe you're seeking something to bring a new dimension of health and wellness into your senior years. Whatever your reason, chair yoga offers a welcoming, gentle, and incredibly effective way to nurture your body and mind.

I discovered the power of chair yoga somewhat serendipitously. As a health and wellness author and practitioner in my mid-forties, I've had the privilege of working with clients of all ages and backgrounds. However, it was my work with seniors that opened my eyes to the unique challenges and opportunities that come with aging. I saw a need for an exercise form that was not only safe and accessible but also enjoyable and beneficial in the long term. That's where chair yoga came in - a practice that respects the body's changes with age and harnesses the timeless principles of yoga to meet these changes with grace, strength, and flexibility.

Chair yoga, as you'll soon discover, is much more than a series of exercises. It's a celebration of what your body can still achieve, a reassurance that age is not a barrier to physical and mental well-being. In this book, you will find exercises designed to improve your strength, mobility, and balance. But more importantly, you will find a practice that brings joy, a sense of achievement, and perhaps a new perspective on what it means to age.

My journey with chair yoga has been as much a learning experience as it has been a teaching one. Each class, each interaction with my wonderful senior students, has taught me something new about resilience, adaptability, and the human spirit's capacity for growth at any age. Their stories of transformation, some of which you will read in this book, are a testament to the power of chair yoga. From regaining the ability to perform everyday tasks with ease to finding a new sense of independence and confidence, these stories are not just inspiring; they are proof of the possibilities that await you.

As we move forward, I encourage you to approach chair yoga with an open heart and mind. This is not a race, nor is it a competition. It's a personal journey, one where progress is measured not by comparison with others but by your own sense of well-being and accomplishment. Whether you are looking to improve your physical health, find mental clarity, or simply add a new dimension to your daily routine, chair yoga can be a rewarding and enriching practice.

In this book, you'll find everything you need to get started on your chair yoga journey. We'll begin with the basics - understanding what chair yoga is, the benefits it offers, and how to practice safely. We'll then move on to more specific routines and exercises, each designed to target different aspects of your physical and mental health. Along the way, I'll be sharing tips, insights, and stories to guide and motivate you.

Remember, this journey is as much about the mind as it is about the body. Chair yoga is not just about physical flexibility and strength;

it's also about cultivating mental resilience, emotional balance, and a deep sense of well-being. As we age, these aspects of health become just as important, if not more so, than physical fitness alone. Through chair yoga, you'll learn not only how to move your body in new and beneficial ways but also how to breathe deeply, focus your mind, and find a sense of calm and centeredness in your day-to-day life.

I invite you to use this book not just as a guide to exercises but as a companion on your journey towards holistic wellness. Take your time with each chapter, listen to your body, and respect its pace. Some days you might feel like challenging yourself a bit more; on others, you might prefer a gentler routine. Chair yoga is flexible and adaptable, just like you.

As we go through this journey together, my hope is that you'll rediscover parts of yourself perhaps forgotten. Maybe it's the strength you thought you had lost, the flexibility you assumed was gone for good, or the balance you've been struggling to find. Chair yoga offers a path to reclaim these qualities, not just in a physical sense but in a way that permeates every aspect of your life.

Your participation in chair yoga is also a powerful statement. It's a declaration that age is not a limitation, that taking care of your body and mind is a priority, and that you're never too old to try something new and transformative. It's about reclaiming your independence, one pose at a time, and embracing the joys and challenges of senior life with a positive, proactive attitude.

In closing this welcome note, I want to express my grati-tude to you, the reader. Thank you for choosing to embark on this journey with me. Your commitment to your health and well-being is inspiring, and I am honored to be a part of it. Together, let's explore the wonderful world of chair yoga and all the benefits it has to offer.

Welcome to the beginning of a beautiful, rewarding journey. Let's start this adventure together, with confidence, curiosity, and a smile.

Warmly,

Laura Garrett

2

—◆—

THE BENEFITS OF CHAIR YOGA

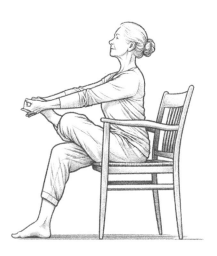

Chair yoga, an innovative adaptation of traditional yoga, of-fers a multitude of health benefits, particularly for seniors. This chapter delves into the scientifically backed advantages of chair yoga, particularly improvements in strength, mobility, balance, and mental health.

Strength Benefits

Chair yoga emerges as an increasingly recognized practice for seniors, particularly for its capacity to mitigate the effects of sarcopenia, the age-related loss of muscle mass and strength. This decline in muscular function, a natural part of the aging process, starts as early as 30 years old and accelerates after the age of 60. The consequences of sarcopenia are profound, including an increased risk of falls, a decline in metabolic rate, and a reduction in the quality of life. However, chair yoga offers a promising countermeasure, providing a safe, accessible, and effective way to build and maintain muscle strength in the senior population.

The strength-building benefits of chair yoga are not just anecdotal but are supported by scientific research. A study conducted by the "International Journal of Yoga Therapy" demonstrated significant improvements in lower-body strength among participants over 60 who engaged in a chair yoga program. These improvements are crucial, considering that lower-body strength is essential for daily activities like walking, climbing stairs, and rising from a seated position.

Chair yoga's effectiveness in combating sarcopenia is rooted in its gentle, low-impact approach to muscle strengthening. Traditional strength-training methods may pose risks for seniors, especially those with limited mobility or chronic conditions. In contrast, chair yoga allows for controlled, mindful movements that target key muscle groups without the strain associated with more rigorous exercise. For instance, chair-based exercises such as seated leg lifts, chair squats, and seated forward bends engage the quadriceps, hamstrings, and core muscles, respectively. These exercises, when performed regularly, contribute to increased muscle mass and improved overall muscular function.

The American Council on Exercise (ACE) underscores the importance of regular strength training for older adults, recommending at least two non-consecutive days per week. Chair yoga fits well within this guideline, providing a structured yet adaptable routine that seniors can follow. The controlled movements in chair yoga, synchronized with breath, allow for a deeper engagement of muscles, leading to more effective strength development. This aspect of controlled movement and breathing also ensures that the exercises are performed safely, reducing the risk of injury.

Furthermore, the progressive nature of chair yoga aligns well with the principles of muscle strengthening. As with any strength training, muscles need to be challenged to grow stronger. Chair yoga allows for this progression; as practitioners become more comfortable and stronger, they can increase the intensity of the movements, add repetitions, or incorporate additional resistance using light weights or resistance bands. This adaptability not only caters to varying levels of physical ability but also ensures that the practice remains challenging and beneficial over time.

Chair yoga also addresses the specific needs of the aging body. As seniors age, joints can become stiffer, and range of motion may decrease. The gentle stretching and strengthening exercises in chair yoga help in maintaining joint health, which is essential for overall muscle function. Improved joint health directly contributes to better muscular control and strength, particularly important for seniors who may be combating arthritis or other joint-related conditions.

Importantly, the benefits of chair yoga in terms of muscle strength extend beyond the exercises themselves. The improvement in muscle strength has a direct correlation with enhanced balance and stability, reducing the likelihood of falls. The Centers for Disease Control and Prevention (CDC) reports that one in four Americans aged 65 and above falls each year, making fall prevention a critical aspect of senior health care. By strengthening the core, hip, and leg muscles, chair yoga significantly contributes to enhancing balance and stability, thus playing a vital role in fall prevention. Stronger muscles mean better support for the body's structure, leading to improved posture and balance, which are key factors in preventing falls among seniors.

The relevance of chair yoga in muscle strengthening is further highlighted by its impact on functional independence. Muscle strength is closely tied to the ability to perform everyday tasks independently. A study in the "Archives of Physical Medicine and Rehabilitation" found that an increase in muscle strength, particularly in the lower body, was associated with a higher likelihood of maintaining functional independence in older adults. Chair yoga, by focusing on strengthening exercises that mimic daily movements, such as seated marches or modified chair lunges, directly contributes to preserving and enhancing this functional independence.

Moreover, chair yoga's approach to muscle strengthening is holistic. It not only works on the major muscle groups but also engages the smaller, stabilizing muscles that are often overlooked in traditional exercise routines. These stabilizing muscles are crucial for maintaining joint alignment and preventing injuries. By engaging these muscles through various chair yoga poses, seniors can enjoy a comprehensive strengthening experience, which translates into improved physical performance and reduced risk of muscle imbalances and related injuries.

In addition to improving overall muscle strength, chair yoga also enhances muscular endurance. Endurance is the ability of muscles to perform repeated contractions over time without fatigue. This aspect of muscle fitness is especially important for seniors, as it affects their ability to engage in prolonged activities and maintain an active lifestyle. Regular chair yoga practice helps in building this endurance, enabling seniors to participate in their daily activities with more ease and less fatigue.

In summary, chair yoga stands out as an ideal exercise regimen for seniors seeking to maintain and enhance muscle strength. Its low-impact, adaptable nature makes it suitable for a wide range of physical abilities, ensuring that everyone, regardless of their fitness level, can benefit from its strength-building potential. By incorporating chair yoga into their regular exercise routine, seniors can effectively combat the effects of sarcopenia, improve their functional independence, and enjoy a higher quality of life. This form of yoga is not just about maintaining strength; it's about empowering seniors to live their later years with vitality, stability, and confidence.

Mobility Benefits

Mobility, defined as the ability to move freely and easily, is essential for performing daily activities and maintaining independence. As individuals age, mobility often declines due to factors like reduced joint flexibility, muscle stiffness, and loss of range of motion. This decline can significantly impact the ease of performing everyday tasks and contribute to a decrease in overall activity levels. Chair yoga offers a targeted approach to combat these age-related challenges by focusing on exercises that enhance mobility, making it an invaluable tool for seniors.

The significance of maintaining mobility in seniors is underscored by statistics and studies emphasizing its impact on quality of life. The American Journal of Public Health reports that 1 in 3 adults over the age of 65 experiences difficulty in walking three city blocks or climbing a flight of stairs. Addressing mobility concerns is not just about maintaining physical function; it's also about preserving independence and preventing the psychological impact of reduced mobility.

Chair yoga, with its gentle, adaptable exercises, specifically targets the factors that influence mobility. By combining stretching and strengthening movements, chair yoga works to increase muscle elasticity, improve joint health, and enhance overall range of motion. These benefits are vital, considering that flexibility tends to decrease with age, affecting the ease of daily activities. For instance, the seated spinal twist in chair yoga helps increase the range of motion in the spine, a common area of stiffness among seniors. Similarly, arm stretches and gentle side bends enhance shoulder and lateral flexibility, crucial for tasks such as reaching for objects.

The impact of chair yoga on joint health is particularly noteworthy. Joints can become stiffer and less flexible as we age, often exacerbated by conditions like arthritis. The Centers for Disease Control and Prevention (CDC) estimates that about 49.6% of adults 65 years or older report doctor-diagnosed arthritis. Chair yoga offers a low-impact exercise option that promotes joint lubrication, essential for maintaining flexibility and reducing discomfort associated with joint stiffness. Movements in chair yoga, such as ankle circles and wrist stretches, directly target joint mobility, enhancing fluidity in movements and reducing the risk of injury.

Moreover, chair yoga aids in improving balance, a key component of mobility. Poor balance can lead to falls, which are a leading cause of injury among seniors. According to the National Council on Aging, an older adult is treated in the emergency room for a fall every 11 seconds. Chair yoga helps improve balance by strengthening the muscles that support the joints, particularly in the lower body, and by enhancing proprioceptive abilities – the body's sense of position in space.

The benefits of chair yoga for mobility extend beyond physical improvements. Enhanced mobility contributes to increased confidence and independence in seniors, encouraging them to engage more actively in daily life and social activities. This increase in activity and social engagement has a ripple effect, improving overall well-being and quality of life.

Mental Health Benefits

Mental health, often overlooked in the discourse on aging, is a critical component of overall well-being. As individuals age, they may face various mental health challenges, including depression, anxiety, and feelings of isolation. Chair yoga, with its holistic approach, offers a valuable tool in mitigating these challenges and enhancing mental health among seniors.

The importance of addressing mental health in seniors cannot be overstated. According to the World Health Organization (WHO), approximately 15% of adults aged 60 and over suffer from a mental disorder. Among these, depression is one of the most prevalent, significantly impacting quality of life. The American Journal of Geriatric Psychiatry reports that depression affects approximately 7% of the older adult population. However, activities such as chair yoga can play a vital role in reducing symptoms of depression and improving overall mental health.

Chair yoga incorporates mindfulness and meditative practices, which are key in managing stress and anxiety. A study in the International Journal of Yoga found that older adults practicing yoga experienced significant reductions in symptoms of depression and anxiety. This is attributed to yoga's focus on deep breathing and present-moment awareness, which foster a sense of calm and mental clarity. The rhythmic breathing exercises common in chair yoga, such as diaphragmatic breathing, have been shown to activate the parasympathetic nervous system, reducing stress and promoting relaxation.

Moreover, chair yoga's emphasis on gentle, mindful movements helps seniors develop a greater sense of body awareness and self-compassion. This heightened body awareness, coupled with the practice of accepting and adapting to the body's limitations, can lead to improved self-esteem and a more positive body image. For seniors, who often face societal pressures regarding aging and physical ability, this aspect of chair yoga can be particularly empowering.

The social aspect of participating in chair yoga classes also contributes significantly to mental health. Loneliness and social isolation are major concerns for the elderly, with the National Academies of Sciences, Engineering, and Medicine reporting that more than one-third of adults aged 45 and older feel lonely, and nearly one-fourth of adults aged 65 and older are considered to be socially isolated. Chair yoga classes provide a community setting where seniors can engage with peers, share experiences, and build social connections. This social interaction is crucial for mental health, as it fosters a sense of belonging and reduces feelings of isolation.

Chair yoga also offers cognitive benefits. Engaging in regular mental and physical activity has been shown to improve cognitive function in seniors. The Alzheimer's Association highlights that regular physical activity, including practices like yoga, can have a protective effect on brain health and may reduce the risk of cognitive decline. Chair yoga, with its combination of physical poses, breath work, and mental focus, challenges the mind and body in a harmonious way, enhancing cognitive abilities such as memory, attention, and problem-solving skills.

In addition to cognitive benefits, chair yoga can improve sleep quality, a common concern among seniors. The National Sleep Foundation notes that 44% of older persons experience one or more symptoms of insomnia. The relaxation and stress-reduction techniques inherent in chair yoga, such as guided relaxation and meditation, can significantly improve sleep patterns. By reducing stress hormones and promoting a state of calm, chair yoga helps in fostering a more restful and rejuvenating sleep, which is essential for mental health and overall well-being.

The impact of chair yoga on mood and emotional well-being is also noteworthy. Engaging in regular yoga practice has been associated with increased levels of serotonin, often referred to as the 'feel-good' neurotransmitter. A study published in the "Journal of Psychiatric Research" found that yoga participants showed significantly higher levels of serotonin and lower levels of monoamine oxidase (an enzyme that breaks down neuro-transmitters), suggesting a positive effect on mood and emotional regulation.

Furthermore, the practice of chair yoga can lead to a decrease in the symptoms of post-traumatic stress disorder (PTSD), which can affect seniors, especially those with a history of significant life traumas or veterans. Research in the "Journal of Traumatic Stress" indicated that yoga, including gentle forms like chair yoga, can reduce symptoms of PTSD, offering a non-invasive and accessible method for managing this condition.

The role of chair yoga in managing chronic pain, which can significantly affect mental health, is also critical. Chronic pain is a common issue among seniors, often leading to a reliance on pain medications, which can have adverse side effects and impact mental clarity. Chair yoga provides a natural, drug-free way to manage pain. The "Annals of Internal Medicine" reported that yoga can be effective in reducing pain and improving function in individuals with chronic back pain, a common ailment in the elderly population.

In summary, chair yoga offers a multifaceted approach to enhancing mental health in seniors. By addressing issues such as depression, anxiety, stress, loneliness, cognitive decline, poor sleep quality, mood fluctuations, PTSD, and chronic pain, chair yoga serves as a comprehensive tool for promoting mental well-being. Its combination of physical movement, breath work, mindfulness, and social interaction makes chair yoga an ideal practice for seniors seeking to improve their mental health and overall quality of life.

3

— • —

SUCCESS STORIES

Jennifer – Healing After A Hip Replacement

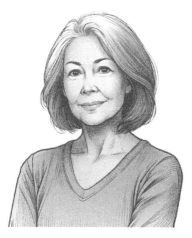

Jennifer, in her late sixties, never thought a hip replacement would be the turning point in her journey towards health and independence. Before the surgery, she led an active life, filled with gardening, long walks with her dog, and playing with her grandchildren. However, things took a sharp turn when her doctor diagnosed her with severe hip osteoarthritis, a condition that gradually eroded her mobility and independence, leading to the inevitable decision of undergoing hip replacement surgery.

The surgery, while successful in alleviating the debilitating pain, brought with it a new set of challenges. Jennifer faced a long road to recovery, marked by physical therapy sessions and a seemingly endless list of restrictions. The experience was not just physically draining but also emotionally taxing. She found herself grappling with a sense of loss – loss of mobility, independence, and a part of her identity.

It was during this period of convalescence that Jennifer discovered chair yoga. Initially skeptical, she was encouraged by her daughter, a yoga enthusiast, to give it a try. Jennifer attended her first chair yoga class with a mix of apprehension and hope, uncertain about what to expect. The class, led by a gentle instructor well-versed in adapting yoga for seniors and individuals with mobility issues, turned out to be a revelation.

Jennifer found that the movements in chair yoga, though gentle, were incredibly effective. The exercises, tailored to suit her condition, focused on slowly rebuilding her strength and flexibility, particularly around her hip. She learned to listen to her body, recognizing its limits and potential. The stretches and poses, once challenging, gradually became easier, and Jennifer began to notice improvements in her mobility and reduction in post-surgical discomfort.

Beyond the physical benefits, chair yoga brought an unexpected gift – a newfound sense of peace and mental clarity. The mindfulness aspect of the practice, which Jennifer initially overlooked, became integral to her recovery. The breathing exercises and meditation techniques taught in her classes helped her manage the anxiety and depression that often accompanied long-term recovery. She found solace in the moments of stillness, a stark contrast to the frustration and restlessness that had previously consumed her days.

Jennifer's commitment to her chair yoga practice deepened over time. She attended classes regularly, slowly becoming a part of the community. The support and encouragement she received from her fellow practitioners and instructor were invaluable. They shared stories, laughter, and, sometimes, frustrations, forming a bond that went beyond the yoga studio.

As weeks turned into months, Jennifer's progress was remarkable. Not only did her physical capabilities improve, but her outlook on life also transformed. She began to reclaim the independence she thought she had lost, engaging more in activities she loved, albeit with a newfound respect for her body's capabilities and limits. Gardening resumed, albeit with more breaks and less strain; walks with her dog became longer and more enjoyable, and playing with her grandchildren was no longer a source of pain but of joy.

Jennifer's journey with chair yoga was not just about physical rehabilitation; it was a journey of emotional and mental resilience. It taught her the importance of patience, the strength of community, and the power of a mindful approach to life's challenges. Her story became a source of inspiration in her chair yoga class, encouraging others facing similar challenges.

In retrospect, Jennifer viewed her hip replacement not just as a medical necessity but as an opportunity that led her to discover chair yoga – a practice that significantly enhanced her quality of life. It was a testament to her resilience and the transformative power of adapting and embracing change, no matter the stage of life.

Jennifer's experience with chair yoga after her hip replacement serves as a compelling success story, highlighting the profound impact of this gentle yet effective practice on recovery, well-being, and overall quality of life for seniors facing health challenges.

Carol – Reducing Her Reliance On A Cane

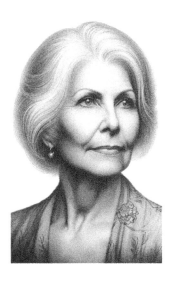

Carol, a vibrant woman in her early seventies, had always cherished her independence. But when age and arthritis began to take their toll, necessitating the use of a cane, she felt as if a part of her freedom was slipping away. The cane, initially a support, gradually became a symbol of her growing limitations. It was during this challenging phase that Carol encountered chair yoga, a practice that would remarkably alter her relationship with her cane and herself.

Before arthritis began to impede her mobility, Carol was an avid walker and an active member of her community. The gradual onset of joint pain and stiffness, particularly in her knees, led to a reluctant but necessary reliance on a cane. This reliance was not just physical; it became an emotional crutch that affected her self-esteem and independence. Carol's world seemed to shrink, her walks became shorter, and her participation in community activities waned.

It was Carol's longtime friend, and fellow walking enthusiast, who first introduced her to chair yoga. The friend, having noticed Carol's increasing dependence on her cane and the subtle changes in her demeanor, suggested they attend a class together. Carol, albeit hesitant, agreed, driven by a mix of curiosity and the faint hope of finding a way to ease her discomfort and regain some of her mobility.

The first chair yoga class was a revelation to Carol. The instructor, with a warm and understanding approach, guided the class through a series of gentle movements and stretches, all performed with the aid of a chair. Carol was surprised at the range of exercises she could perform despite her limitations. The classes emphasized strengthening and stretching, particularly around the joints, which was exactly what Carol needed.

Over time, Carol began to notice significant improvements. The exercises helped alleviate some of her joint stiffness, making movement easier and less painful. She found herself relying less on her cane within her home, using it only for longer walks or outings. The most profound change, however, was in her sense of self. Chair yoga helped Carol reconnect with her body in a compassionate way, teaching her to recognize and work within her limits without feeling defeated by them.

More than the physical benefits, chair yoga brought a mental transformation. The mindfulness and breathing techniques practiced in class helped Carol manage the frustration and sadness associated with her physical limitations. She learned to approach her condition with a sense of acceptance and grace, rather than resistance and despair. This shift in mindset was instrumental in her journey towards reduced reliance on her cane.

As Carol continued with chair yoga, her confidence grew. She began to participate more actively in her community, no longer feeling sidelined by her physical constraints. The cane, which once felt like a tether, now became just another tool she occasionally used, no longer a symbol of her limitations but a testament to her resilience.

Carol's journey with chair yoga is a story of empowerment. It demonstrates how adapting and finding alternative ways to stay active can significantly impact physical ability and mental well-being. Her reduced reliance on the cane was not just a physical achievement but also a symbol of her regained independence and renewed spirit.

Carol's success story with chair yoga stands as an inspiration to others facing similar challenges. It underscores the power of gentle, consistent exercise and the profound impact of a positive, accepting mindset in overcoming life's obstacles.

George – Going Back to Golfing

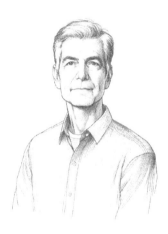

George, in his late seventies, had always found solace and joy on the golf course. It was more than a sport for him; it was a ritual, a cherished weekly tradition that connected him to friends and nature. However, as the years progressed, George began to experience a decline in his mobility and balance, a change that deeply affected his golf game. The sport that once brought him so much pleasure became a source of frustration, as he struggled with the physical demands it required. The turning point in his journey came when he discovered chair yoga, a practice that not only rejuvenated his love for golf but also restored his ability to play.

For George, the challenges on the golf course began subtly - a decrease in swing range, difficulty in maintaining balance, and a gradual increase in post-game fatigue and discomfort. These issues didn't just affect his performance; they started to erode his confidence. Golf, which had always been a source of joy and pride, became a reminder of his aging body's limitations. It was during a particularly disheartening round of golf that a friend, noticing George's struggles, suggested chair yoga. Skeptical but desperate to find a solution, George decided to give it a try.

Attending his first chair yoga class, George was immediately struck by the welcoming atmosphere and the instructor's understanding of the physical challenges faced by seniors. The class focused on gentle yet effective exercises that targeted balance, flexibility, and core strength - all key components crucial for a golfer. George was surprised at how the movements and stretches, though performed in a chair, mimicked the motions used in golf, particularly the twisting and turning of the torso.

As George incorporated chair yoga into his weekly routine, he began to notice significant improvements. His balance improved markedly, a change that translated directly to a more stable and powerful golf swing. The flexibility exercises enhanced his range of motion, allowing him to execute a fuller swing with less discomfort. Perhaps most importantly, the core-strengthening aspects of chair yoga provided him with better control and power in his shots.

Beyond the physical benefits, chair yoga offered George mental and emotional gains. The mindfulness and breathing techniques learned in class helped him maintain focus and composure on the golf course, especially under pressure. He found himself more present in each moment of the game, enjoying the experience regardless of the outcome of each shot.

Gradually, George's performance on the golf course transformed. He was hitting the ball further, experiencing less fatigue, and most importantly, enjoying the game again. His renewed ability and confidence were noticed by his golfing buddies, who marveled at the improvement in his game. George's story became a topic of conversation at the clubhouse, inspiring other senior golfers to consider chair yoga as a means to enhance their own game.

For George, chair yoga was more than just a set of exercises; it was a pathway to reclaiming a part of his life that he thought he had lost. It allowed him to reconnect with his passion for golf, not just by improving his physical abilities but also by instilling a sense of resilience and adaptability. George's journey is a testament to the idea that with the right approach and attitude, it's possible to continue enjoying one's passions, regardless of age.

George's success story with chair yoga and golf stands as an inspiring example for seniors facing similar challenges. It highlights the importance of maintaining physical activity and the profound impact it can have on quality of life and the pursuit of lifelong passions.

4

WARM-UP ROUTINES

W arm-up routines serve several crucial functions. Firstly, they gradually increase the heart rate and circulation, sending more oxygen and nutrients to the muscles. This is particularly important for seniors, as their circulatory systems can be less efficient compared to younger adults. A study published in the "Journal of Aging and Physical Activity" found that a proper warm-up improves blood flow to the muscles in older adults, reducing the risk of muscle strain and injuries.

Additionally, warm-ups play a pivotal role in increasing muscle temperature. Warmer muscles are more flexible and less prone to strains. The American Council on Exercise (ACE) notes that proper warm-ups can increase muscle temperature by 1 to 2 degrees, enhancing muscle elasticity and overall performance. For seniors practicing chair yoga, this translates to a reduced risk of pulling or tearing muscles during the session.

Another key benefit of warm-ups is the enhancement of joint mobility. As we age, our joints can become stiffer and less fluid in their movements. Warm-up exercises, particularly those involving gentle joint rotations and stretches, lubricate the joints by increasing the production of synovial fluid. This is crucial for maintaining joint health and preventing injuries such as sprains or joint strains.

Warm-ups also prepare the nervous system for exercise. Gentle, repetitive movements signal the brain to start coordinating with the muscles, improving overall movement efficiency and reaction time. For seniors, whose neuromuscular efficiency may have declined with age, this aspect of warm-ups is particularly beneficial. It helps in reducing the risk of falls and other accidents that can occur due to a lack of coordination or delayed reaction times. The National Institute on Aging emphasizes the importance of balance and coordination exercises in preventing falls, which are a leading cause of injury among older adults.

Mentally, warm-ups are just as important. They provide a transition period from rest to exercise, helping to mentally prepare for the yoga practice. This mental preparation is key in fostering a mindful, focused approach to the yoga session. It allows individuals to center themselves, set intentions for their practice, and become more attuned to their body's needs and limitations. A study in the "Journal of Behavioral Medicine" suggests that a proper warm-up can also reduce anxiety and improve concentration, both of which are crucial for a successful chair yoga session.

The risks of skipping warm-ups are significant, especially for seniors. Without adequately preparing the body, jumping straight into a yoga routine can lead to muscle strains, joint pain, and increased susceptibility to injuries. Cold muscles and joints are less flexible and more prone to tears and strains. A report from the "Journal of Sports Science & Medicine" indicates that inadequate warm-up is a common factor in exercise-related injuries in older adults. These injuries can range from minor strains to more serious injuries that could significantly impact mobility and independence.

Specific injuries that can result from inadequate warm-up include muscle tears, tendon strains, ligament sprains, and joint injuries. For example, starting a chair yoga routine without warming up could lead to a hamstring strain or knee joint pain, especially if the routine involves stretches or movements that put a strain on these areas. Additionally, for seniors with existing health conditions like arthritis, failing to warm up properly can exacerbate pain and stiffness in the affected joints.

In summary, warm-up routines are an integral part of chair yoga, especially for seniors. They serve to increase blood flow, improve muscle and joint flexibility, enhance neuromuscular coordination, and prepare the mind for the yoga session. The benefits of a proper warm-up are clear: reduced risk of injury, improved performance, and a more enjoyable yoga experience. Conversely, skipping the warm-up phase can lead to a range of injuries, negatively impacting the overall effectiveness of the yoga practice and the well-being of the practitioner.

In the following sections, we will explore various warm-up exercises and techniques that are ideal for seniors embarking on a chair yoga routine. These exercises will be designed to prepare the body and mind effectively, ensuring a safe and rewarding chair yoga experience.

Breath Work

In chair yoga, breathing exercises form a crucial component of the warm-up routine, preparing both the body and mind for the yoga session. Proper breathing techniques can significantly enhance the effectiveness of the yoga practice, improving oxygenation, reducing stress, and increasing mindfulness. Here, we explore five essential breathing warm-up techniques, each complete with a description, step-by-step guide, and recommended duration.

1. Diaphragmatic Breathing

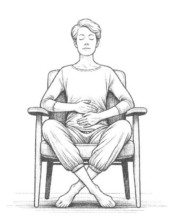

Description:
Diaphragmatic breathing, often called abdominal or belly

breathing, involves deep breathing using the diaphragm muscle. This technique enhances lung capacity and promotes relaxation.

Step-by-Step Guide:

1. Sit comfortably in your chair with your back straight.

2. Place one hand on your abdomen and the other on your chest.

3. Inhale slowly through your nose, feeling your abdomen expand while keeping your chest relatively still.

4. Exhale slowly through your mouth or nose, feeling your abdomen fall.

5. Repeat this process, focusing on deep, full breaths.

Duration:

Practice for 3-5 minutes.

2. Three-Part Breath

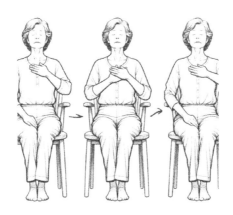

Description:

The Three-Part Breath, or Dirga Pranayama, involves dividing the breath into three parts, sequentially filling the abdomen, diaphragm, and chest.

Step-by-Step Guide:

1. Sit upright in your chair, relaxing your shoulders.

2. Begin by inhaling deeply, filling your lower belly, then your ribcage, and finally your upper chest.

3. Exhale in reverse order: chest, ribcage, and lower belly.

4. Use your hands to feel each section of your torso rise and fall as you breathe.

5. Focus on making each of the three parts of the breath
   smooth and fluid.

Duration:

Continue for 4-6 minutes.

3. Alternate Nostril Breathing

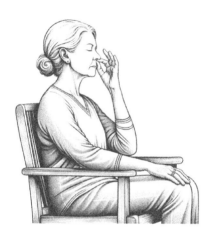

Description:

Alternate Nostril Breathing, or Nadi Shodhana, is a technique that involves alternating the breath between the nostrils. This practice balances the left and right hemispheres of the brain and calms the mind.

Step-by-Step Guide:

1. Sit comfortably with your spine erect.

2. Place your left hand on your left knee.

3. Use your right thumb to close your right nostril and inhale deeply through your left nostril.

4. Close your left nostril with your right ring finger, open

your right nostril, and exhale.

5. Inhale through the right nostril, close it, and exhale through the

left nostril.

6. This completes one cycle. Continue alternating between each nostril, focusing on smooth and even breaths.

Duration:

Practice for 5-7 minutes.

4. Ujjayi Breath

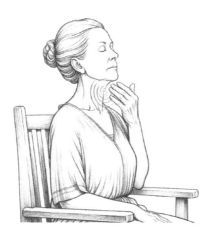

Description:

Ujjayi Breath, also known as the "Ocean Breath" or "Victorious Breath," involves a slight constriction of the back of the throat to create a gentle sound as you breathe. This technique enhances focus and presence.

Step-by-Step Guide:

1. Sit comfortably with your spine straight.

2. Inhale deeply through your nose.

3. As you exhale, slightly constrict the back of your throat and make a soft hissing sound, similar to the sound of the ocean.

4. Keep this constriction both during inhales and exhales, focusing on the sound and rhythm of your breath.

5. Ensure your breathing is slow and rhythmic.

Duration:

Engage in this breath for 4-6 minutes.

5. Bee Breath

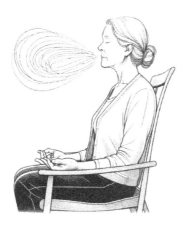

Description:

Bee Breath, or Bhramari Pranayama, involves making a humming sound during exhalation. This technique is effective for calming the mind and relieving stress or anxiety.

Step-by-Step Guide:

1. Sit straight and relaxed in your chair.

2. Close your eyes and take a few normal breaths to settle in.

3. Place your index fingers on the cartilage between your cheek and ear.

4. Inhale deeply through your nose.

5. As you exhale, gently press the cartilage while making a humming sound like a bee.

6. Feel the vibration of the sound in your head.

7. Repeat the process, focusing on the humming sound and vibration.

Duration:

Practice for 5-7 minutes.

Each of these breathing techniques serves as a gentle warm-up for the respiratory system, preparing the body for physical activity while calming the mind and enhancing mental focus. By incorporating these breathing exercises into the beginning of a chair yoga session, practitioners can significantly improve their overall yoga experience, ensuring they are mentally and physically ready for the poses and stretches to follow.

Warm-Up Stretches

Stretching, at its core, is about improving flexibility – the ability of the muscles and joints to move through their full range of motion. As we age, our bodies naturally lose some of this flexibility due to changes in muscle and connective tissue. This loss can lead to a decrease in mobility, increased discomfort during movement, and a higher risk of injury. Regular stretching, however, can mitigate these age-related changes, maintaining or even enhancing flexibility.

The significance of maintaining flexibility in older adults is well-documented. Research in the "Journal of Aging and Physical Activity" shows that enhanced flexibility contributes to better functional movement, making daily tasks like reaching, bending, or walking more comfortable and safer. Stretching the muscles regularly keeps them long, lean, and flexible, reducing the stiffness and pain that can impede everyday activities.

Beyond flexibility, stretching plays a critical role in injury prevention. Tight muscles are more prone to strains and tears, as they are unable to absorb sudden movements or stresses as effectively as supple muscles. This is particularly important for seniors, who may be more susceptible to injuries due to decreased bone density and muscle mass. A study in the "American Journal of Sports Medicine" found that a routine of regular stretching significantly reduces the risk of injury in older adults by maintaining muscle and joint health.

Furthermore, stretching has a notable impact on posture. Poor posture, common in older adults due to factors like muscle weakness and gravitational changes, can lead to discomfort and health issues such as back pain and impaired digestion. Stretching the muscles of the back, shoulders, and chest helps counteract these postural changes, promoting a more upright and aligned posture. Improved posture not only reduces the risk of pain and injury but also enhances breathing and circulation.

The benefits of stretching also extend to overall physical and mental well-being. Engaging in a regular stretching routine has been shown to increase blood flow to the muscles, providing them with more oxygen and nutrients while removing waste products. This enhanced circulation can lead to increased energy levels and improved overall health. Moreover, stretching, especially when combined with mindful breathing as in chair yoga, can be a powerful stress-reliever. The "International Journal of Yoga" highlights the calming effects of stretching combined with deep breathing, noting reductions in stress and anxiety levels among practitioners.

For seniors practicing chair yoga, stretching also provides an opportunity to connect with their bodies in a nurturing and respectful way. It encourages mindfulness and body awareness, allowing practitioners to tune into their physical needs and limitations. This mindful approach to movement can foster a deeper sense of body acceptance and self-care, important aspects of mental and emotional health in the senior years.

1. Seated Side Stretch

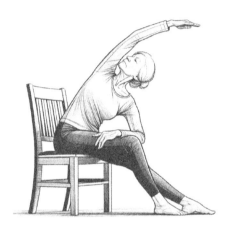

Description:

The Seated Side Stretch elongates the side muscles, improves lateral flexibility, and helps open up the ribcage for better breathing.

Step-by-Step Guide:

1. Sit upright in your chair with feet flat on the ground.

2. Extend your right arm overhead and lean to your left side, keeping your left hand on your left thigh.

3. Feel the stretch along the right side of your body.

4. Hold for a few breaths, then return to the starting position.

5. Repeat on the left side.

Duration:

Hold each side for 20-30 seconds. Repeat 2-3 times on each side.

2. Forward Bend

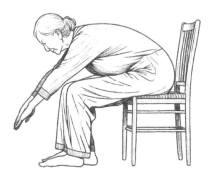

Description:

The Forward Bend stretches the spine, shoulders, and hamstrings, and can relieve tension in the back and neck.

Step-by-Step Guide:

1. Sit on the edge of your chair with your feet slightly apart.

2. Inhale and extend your arms overhead.

3. Exhale and slowly bend forward from your hips, lowering your hands towards your feet.

4. Let your head and neck relax.

5. Hold the stretch, then slowly rise back to the starting position.

Duration:

Hold the position for 20-30 seconds. Repeat 2-3 times.

3. Neck Stretch

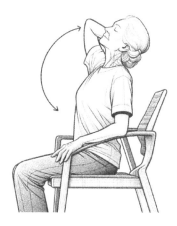

Description:

The Neck Stretch targets the muscles in the neck, helping to relieve tension and improve flexibility in this often-stiff area.

Step-by-Step Guide:

1. Sit comfortably in your chair with your feet flat on the floor and your hands resting on your lap.

2. Gently tilt your head towards your right shoulder, bringing your ear closer to the shoulder.

3. To deepen the stretch, you can gently press down on your head with your right hand.

4. Hold the position, feeling the stretch on the left side of

your neck.

5. Slowly return to the center and repeat on the left side.

Duration:

Hold each side for 20-30 seconds. Repeat 2-3 times on each side.

4. Seated Cat-Cow Stretch

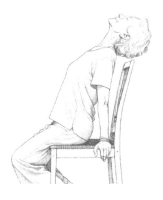

Description:

The Seated Cat-Cow Stretch is a gentle movement that improves flexibility in the spine and helps relieve tension in the back and neck.

Step-by-Step Guide:

1. Sit at the edge of your chair with your feet flat on the ground and hands on your knees.

2. Inhale, arch your back and look up towards the ceiling, pushing your chest forward (Cow position).

3. Exhale, round your spine, tuck in your chin to your chest, and bring your belly towards your spine (Cat

position).

4. Continue this movement, flowing from Cat to Cow, and back again.

Duration:

Perform this movement for 1-2 minutes.

5. Seated Spinal Twist

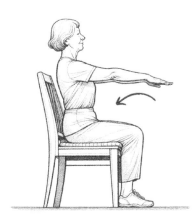

Description:

The Seated Spinal Twist increases spinal mobility, stretches the back muscles, and can aid in digestion and circulation.

Step-by-Step Guide:

1. Sit sideways on your chair, facing to the right.

2. Keep your feet flat on the floor and align your knees.

3. Twist your torso to the right, holding onto the back of the chair for support.

4. Hold the twist, feeling the stretch in your spine and back.

5. Slowly release and turn your body to face the left side of the chair, repeating the twist on the other side.

Duration:

Hold each twist for 20-30 seconds. Repeat 2-3 times on each side.

5

MOBILITY EXERCISES

As the body ages, natural changes occur in the joints, muscles, and connective tissues, leading to decreased flexibility and mobility. According to the American College of Rheumatology, more than half of seniors over the age of 65 experience some degree of joint stiffness and reduced mobility. This reduction in mobility can significantly impact daily activities, making simple tasks like reaching for objects, bending, or walking challenging. Furthermore, reduced mobility is closely linked to an increased risk of falls, a major concern for seniors. The Centers for Disease Control and Prevention (CDC) reports that falls are the leading cause of injury and injury-related death among adults aged 65 and older.

Chair yoga, with its gentle, adaptable exercises, serves as an ideal solution for improving mobility in seniors. By focusing on movements that enhance joint flexibility and increase the range of motion, chair yoga helps mitigate the effects of aging on the body. These exercises promote the production of synovial fluid, lubricating the joints and reducing stiffness. Improved joint health directly translates into better mobility, making daily movements smoother and less painful.

In addition to joint health, chair yoga exercises also target muscle flexibility. As per the National Institute on Aging, maintaining muscle flexibility is essential for balance, posture, and overall functional ability. Chair yoga includes stretches and poses that lengthen and strengthen the muscles, enhancing flexibility and reducing the risk of muscle strains or injury.

The benefits of improved mobility through chair yoga extend beyond physical health. A study in the "Journal of Aging Research" found that increased mobility leads to better overall quality of life and reduced feelings of depression and isolation among seniors. Mobility is closely linked to independence, a crucial aspect of well-being for older adults. The ability to move freely and perform daily tasks without assistance fosters a sense of autonomy and self-confidence.

Moreover, enhanced mobility contributes to social engagement and active living. Seniors with better mobility are more likely to participate in community activities, engage in social interactions, and maintain an active lifestyle. The "Journal of Gerontology" reported that seniors with higher mobility levels experience more frequent social interactions, which are vital for mental and emotional health.

Chair yoga mobility exercises are designed to be accessible, allowing seniors of varying physical abilities to participate. These exercises can be modified to suit individual needs, ensuring that everyone can benefit from the practice regardless of their starting level of flexibility or mobility.

The importance of mobility for seniors cannot be overstated. It is a key factor in maintaining independence, preventing falls, and enjoying a high quality of life. Chair yoga offers a gentle yet effective way to enhance mobility, addressing the specific needs of the aging body. Through regular practice, seniors can enjoy greater freedom of movement, reduced pain, and an overall sense of well-being.

In this section, we will explore five essential mobility exercises in chair yoga. Each exercise is described in detail, with a step-by-step guide and recommended duration, providing seniors with practical tools to improve their mobility and enhance their quality of life.

1. Seated Knee Lifts

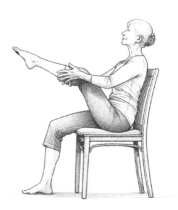

Description:

Seated knee lifts focus on enhancing hip mobility and strengthening the lower abdomen and thigh muscles.

Step-by-Step Guide:

1. Sit upright in your chair, feet flat on the floor, hands resting on your thighs.

2. Slowly lift your right knee towards your chest, keeping your back straight.

3. Hold your knee with both hands for a deeper stretch.

4. Gently lower your leg back to the starting position.

5. Repeat with your left leg.

Duration:

Do 8-10 lifts per leg, repeating for 2-3 sets.

2. Ankle Circles

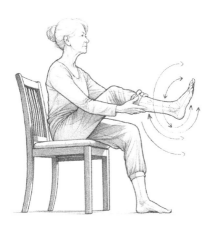

Description:

Ankle circles improve ankle mobility and flexibility, reducing stiffness and aiding in balance.

Step-by-Step Guide:

1. Sit in your chair with your feet flat on the ground.

2. Extend one leg out in front of you, keeping the heel on the floor.

3. Slowly rotate your ankle clockwise for several circles, then counter-clockwise.

4. Lower your leg and repeat with the other ankle.

Duration:

Perform 10 circles in each direction per ankle.

3. Seated Hip Openers

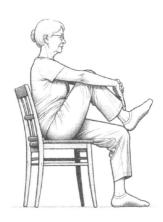

Description:

Seated hip openers target the hip joints and inner thighs, areas prone to stiffness in seniors.

Step-by-Step Guide:

1. Sit upright in your chair, feet flat on the floor.

2. Place your right ankle on your left knee, forming a figure-four shape.

3. Gently press down on your right knee for a deeper hip stretch.

4. Hold the position, then slowly release and switch legs.

Duration:

Hold each stretch for 20-30 seconds. Repeat 2-3 times on each side.

4. Chair Pigeon Pose

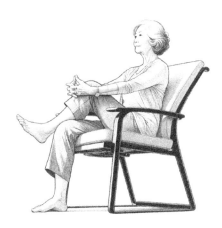

Description:

The Chair Pigeon Pose stretches the hip flexors, glutes, and lower back, essential for lower body mobility.

Step-by-Step Guide:

1. Sit at the edge of your chair, feet flat on the ground.

2. Cross your right ankle over your left thigh, keeping your knee in line with your ankle.

3. Lean forward slightly from your hips, maintaining a straight back.

4. Hold the stretch, then slowly come back up and switch sides.

Duration:

Hold for 20-30 seconds per side, repeating 2-3 times.

5. Spinal Rotation

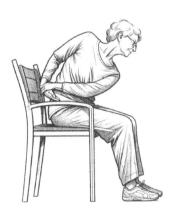

Description:

Spinal rotation enhances flexibility in the spine and shoulders, crucial for upper body mobility.

Step-by-Step Guide:

1. Sit upright in your chair, feet flat on the floor, hands on your knees.

2. As you inhale, lengthen your spine.

3. As you exhale, gently twist your torso to the right, placing your left hand on your right knee and your right hand behind you.

4. Hold the twist, then slowly return to center and repeat

on the left side.

Duration:

Twist and hold for 15-20 seconds on each side. Repeat 2-3 times.

Each of these mobility exercises in chair yoga is specifically tailored to address the common areas of stiffness and limited movement in seniors. They are designed to be gentle yet effective, ensuring that practitioners can safely enhance their mobility without the risk of strain or injury.

The Seated Knee Lifts focus on the hips, a crucial joint that affects walking, sitting, and standing. Improved hip mobility can lead to better balance and reduced risk of falls. Ankle Circles are vital for maintaining ankle flexibility, which is essential for stable walking and standing. This exercise also helps in preventing conditions like ankle stiffness or swelling, common in less active seniors.

Seated Hip Openers and Chair Pigeon Pose target the hip flexors and glutes, areas that often become tight due to prolonged sitting or lack of activity. These stretches are particularly beneficial for alleviating lower back pain, a common complaint among older adults. Regularly practicing these exercises can significantly improve the range of motion in the hips, enhancing the ability to perform daily activities like bending and squatting with greater ease.

The Spinal Rotation exercise is key for maintaining spinal health. The spine's flexibility is essential for various movements, from turning to look behind to reaching for objects. This exercise not only improves spinal mobility but also helps in relieving tension in the back muscles, enhancing overall posture.

Incorporating these mobility exercises into a regular chair yoga routine can have profound benefits for seniors. Improved joint flexibility and range of motion can lead to a more active lifestyle, greater independence, and enhanced overall well-being. These exercises also promote better circulation, which is essential for muscle health and injury prevention.

Furthermore, the focus on gentle movement helps in building body awareness and mindfulness. Seniors become more attuned to their bodies, learning to move in ways that are beneficial and not harmful, fostering a deeper connection between the mind and body. This mindful approach to movement can have positive effects on mental health as well, reducing stress and promoting a sense of calm.

6

STRENGTH EXERCISES

S trength training, often overshadowed by cardiovascular and flexibility exercises, holds paramount importance in the overall health regimen of seniors. This 800-word section delves into the myriad benefits of strength training for older adults, emphasizing its necessity through quantifiable data and research findings.

As individuals age, they naturally experience a decline in muscle mass and strength, a condition known as sarcopenia. According to a study published in the "Journal of Cachexia, Sarcopenia and Muscle," sarcopenia affects approximately 10% of adults over the age of 60. This muscle loss significantly impacts daily activities, increases the risk of falls and injuries, and can lead to a decline in overall quality of life. However, strength training emerges as a powerful tool to counteract these effects. Regular strength training can not only slow down the loss of muscle mass but can also rebuild strength, even in individuals who begin exercising later in life.

The benefits of strength training extend beyond muscle health. A study in the "Journal of the American Geriatrics Society" found that older adults who engage in regular strength training have a 23% reduction in the risk of all-cause mortality compared to those who do not. This underscores the vital role of muscle strengthening in promoting longevity and overall health.

One significant benefit of strength training for seniors is the improvement in functional independence. Activities such as carrying groceries, climbing stairs, or even getting up from a chair become more manageable with increased muscle strength. The "Archives of Physical Medicine and Rehabilitation" reports that strength training improves functional performance in older adults, thereby enhancing their ability to perform everyday tasks and maintain independence.

Strength training also plays a crucial role in managing and preventing chronic diseases. The American Heart Association highlights that regular muscle-strengthening activities can help control blood sugar levels, an essential factor for managing or preventing type 2 diabetes. Additionally, strength training is beneficial for bone health. The National Osteoporosis Foundation advocates for strength training exercises to maintain and improve bone density, crucial for preventing osteoporosis, a condition that affects over 200 million people worldwide.

Falls are a leading cause of injury among seniors, and strength training can significantly reduce this risk. The Centers for Disease Control and Prevention (CDC) report that one in four

Americans aged 65 and over falls each year. Strength training enhances balance and stability, making falls less likely. A study in the "Journal of Gerontology" found that strength training reduced the rate of falls by 40% among participants aged 65 and older.

In addition to physical benefits, strength training has a positive impact on mental health. Regular participation in strength training activities has been linked to reductions in symptoms of depression and anxiety. The "American Journal of Epidemiology" found that older adults who engaged in regular strength training had a 20% lower risk of developing depression. The mental stimulation and sense of achievement associated with strength training also contribute to improved cognitive function. Research in the "Archives of Internal Medicine" suggests that older adults who engage in strength training experience slower cognitive decline.

Moreover, strength training is instrumental in weight management. As metabolism naturally slows with age, maintaining a healthy weight can become more challenging. Muscle tissue burns more calories than fat tissue, even at rest. Therefore, building muscle through strength training can increase metabolic rate, aiding in weight control. The "Obesity" journal reports that strength training is effective in reducing body fat and increasing lean muscle mass in older adults.

1. Seated Leg Extensions

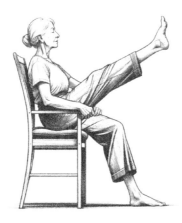

Description:

Seated leg extensions strengthen the quadriceps, the muscles at the front of the thigh, essential for walking and standing activities.

Step-by-Step Guide:

1. Sit upright in a chair with feet flat on the floor.

2. Extend one leg out in front of you as straight as possible.

3. Flex your foot to engage the muscles in your leg.

4. Hold the extension for a few seconds, then lower your leg back down.

5. Repeat with the other leg.

Duration:

Do 10-15 extensions per leg, for 2-3 sets.

2. Chair Squats

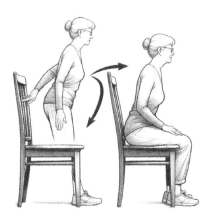

Description:

Chair squats target the glutes, quadriceps, and hamstrings, improving lower body strength and balance.

Step-by-Step Guide:

1. Start by sitting in a chair with your feet shoulder-width apart.

2. Lean slightly forward and stand up from the chair.

3. Slowly lower yourself back into the chair, controlling the movement.

4. Keep your weight on your heels and your knees aligned with your feet.

Duration:

Perform 10-12 squats, for 2-3 sets.

3. Arm Raises

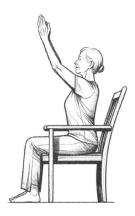

Description:

Arm raises strengthen the shoulders and improve upper body mobility, important for tasks like lifting objects.

Step-by-Step Guide:

1. Sit upright with your arms at your sides and palms facing down.

2. Slowly raise your arms to the side or front, up to shoulder height.

3. Hold for a moment, then lower your arms back down.

4. Keep your movements slow and controlled.

Duration:

Do 10-15 arm raises, for 2-3 sets.

4. Seated Rows

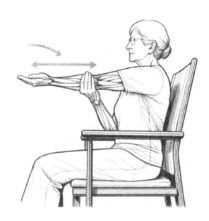

Description:

Seated rows focus on the upper back and shoulder muscles, crucial for posture and upper body strength.

Step-by-Step Guide:

1. Sit upright with your feet flat on the ground.

2. Extend your arms in front of you, then pull your elbows back, squeezing your shoulder blades together.

3. Return your arms to the extended position and repeat.

4. Imagine you are pulling against resistance to engage your muscles more.

Duration:

Complete 10-15 rows, for 2-3 sets.

5. Seated Tummy Twists

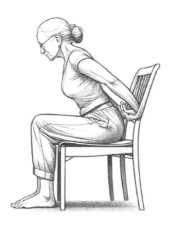

Description:

Seated tummy twists strengthen the core muscles, which are vital for balance and spinal support.

Step-by-Step Guide:

1. Sit on the edge of your chair with your feet flat on the floor.

2. Place your hands behind your head, elbows wide.

3. Gently twist your torso to the right, then to the left, engaging your abdominal muscles.

4. Keep your movements slow and controlled, focusing on the twist.

Duration:

Do 10-12 twists to each side, for 2-3 sets.

7

MINDFULNESS EXERCISES

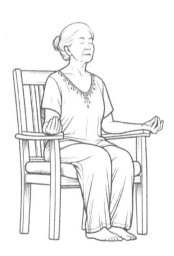

Mindfulness meditation involves paying deliberate attention to the present moment, acknowledging and accepting one's thoughts, feelings, and bodily sensations without judgment. This form of meditation, rooted in Buddhist traditions, has been adapted and popularized in Western cultures as a tool for reducing stress, improving mental clarity, and enhancing overall well-being.

For seniors, the practice of mindfulness meditation is of immense value. As we age, we often face a variety of challenges, including health issues, loss of loved ones, and changes in social roles. Mindfulness meditation offers a way to navigate these changes with greater ease and resilience. A study in the "Journal of Applied Gerontology" found that mindfulness meditation can significantly reduce feelings of loneliness in older adults, a key factor contributing to various physical and mental health issues.

One of the primary benefits of mindfulness meditation is stress reduction. Seniors, grappling with the challenges of aging, can find themselves under significant stress, which can exacerbate health problems and impair cognitive function. Mindfulness meditation has been shown to reduce the production of stress hormones, such as cortisol. Research published in the "Health Psychology" journal reported a notable decrease in cortisol levels among participants engaged in regular mindfulness practices. This reduction in stress can lead to lower blood pressure, reduced risk of heart disease, and a better overall quality of life.

Mindfulness meditation also has substantial mental health benefits. It has been effectively used as a tool in treating depression and anxiety, common among seniors. According to a study in the "Journal of Psychiatric Practice," mindfulness-based interventions can lead to significant reductions in symptoms of depression and anxiety. By fostering a practice of present-moment awareness and acceptance, mindfulness meditation helps break the cycle of negative thoughts, a common feature of depression and anxiety disorders.

Additionally, mindfulness meditation can enhance cognitive function in older adults. With age comes the risk of cognitive decline, including memory loss and decreased concentration. Mindfulness practices have been found to improve attention, clarity of thought, and emotional regulation. A study in the "Journal of Alzheimer's Disease" indicated that mindfulness meditation could slow the progression of cognitive decline, particularly in those at risk for developing Alzheimer's disease.

Another significant benefit of mindfulness meditation for seniors is pain management. Chronic pain is a common issue in the elderly, often leading to a reliance on pain medications. Mindfulness meditation offers a natural, non-pharmacological approach to managing pain. According to research in the "Clinical Journal of Pain," mindfulness-based stress reduction techniques were effective in reducing chronic pain symptoms and improving quality of life among older adults.

Furthermore, mindfulness meditation fosters a greater sense of connectedness and empathy, which can be especially beneficial for seniors who may experience feelings of isolation or disconnection. Engaging in mindfulness practices can enhance emotional intelligence and improve interpersonal relationships. The "American Journal of Geriatric Psychiatry" highlights that mindfulness interventions can improve emotional well-being and social interactions in older adults.

In the realm of physical health, mindfulness meditation has been linked to improved immune function. A study in the "Psychosomatic Medicine" journal reported that mindfulness meditation could boost the immune response, leading to a better defense against illnesses. This is particularly crucial for seniors, who may have weakened immune systems.

1. Mindful Breathing

Description:

Mindful breathing involves focusing on the breath, a fundamental exercise in mindfulness meditation.

Step-by-Step Guide:

1. Sit comfortably in a quiet space.

2. Close your eyes and take a few deep breaths.

3. Shift your attention to your natural breathing pattern.

4. Notice the sensation of air entering and leaving your nostrils.

5. If your mind wanders, gently bring it back to your breath.

6. Continue for 5-10 minutes.

2. Body Scan Meditation

Description:

Body scan meditation promotes awareness of bodily sensations and helps release tension.

Step-by-Step Guide:

1. Lie down or sit comfortably.

2. Close your eyes and take deep breaths.

3. Focus on your feet, noticing any sensations.

4. Gradually move your attention up through each part of your body.

5. If you notice tension, imagine it melting away.

6. Continue until you reach the top of your head.

7. Finish with a few deep breaths.

3. Walking Meditation

Description:

Walking meditation combines mindfulness with gentle physical activity.

Step-by-Step Guide:

1. Find a quiet place to walk.

2. Focus on the sensation of your feet touching the ground.

3. Walk slowly, paying attention to the movement of your legs.

4. If your mind wanders, gently redirect it to your walking.

5. Continue for 10-15 minutes.

4. Mindful Eating

Description:

Mindful eating is about experiencing food more intensely and eating consciously.

Step-by-Step Guide:

1. Choose a small item of food, like a fruit.

2. Look at it carefully, observing its colors and textures.

3. Smell the food and notice any saliva in your mouth.

4. Take a small bite, chew slowly, and savor the taste.

5. Continue eating slowly, focusing on each bite.

5. Gratitude Meditation

Description:

Gratitude meditation involves focusing on things you are thankful for.

Step-by-Step Guide:

1. Sit in a quiet and comfortable place.

2. Think of three things you are grateful for.

3. Reflect on why each thing makes you grateful.

4. Feel the emotions associated with gratitude.

5. End with a few deep breaths, savoring the feeling.

6. Loving-Kindness Meditation

Description:

Loving-kindness meditation fosters a sense of compassion and love for oneself and others.

Step-by-Step Guide:

1. Sit comfortably and close your eyes.

2. Start by directing love and kindness towards yourself.

3. Gradually extend these feelings towards family, friends, and even strangers.

4. Repeat phrases like, "May I/you be happy, may I/you be healthy."

5. Continue for 5-10 minutes.

7. Focused Attention Meditation

Description:

Focused attention meditation involves concentrating on a single object or thought.

Step-by-Step Guide:

1. Choose an object of focus, like a candle flame.

2. Sit comfortably and gaze at the object.

3. Keep your attention on the object, observing every detail.

4. If your mind wanders, gently bring it back to the object.

5. Continue for 5-10 minutes.

8. Sound Meditation

Description:

Sound meditation uses ambient sounds to foster mindfulness.

Step-by-Step Guide:

1. Find a comfortable sitting position.

2. Close your eyes and focus on the sounds around you.

3. Observe each sound without judgment or analysis.

4. Let the sounds come and go naturally.

5. Continue for 10-15 minutes.

9. Visualization Meditation

Description:

Visualization meditation involves picturing a peaceful scene in your mind.

Step-by-Step Guide:

1. Sit or lie down in a comfortable position.

2. Close your eyes and imagine a serene setting.

3. Engage all your senses to bring the scene to life.

4. Allow yourself to feel relaxed and peaceful.

5. Continue for 5-10 minutes.

10. Mindful Movement

Description:

Mindful movement combines gentle physical exercises with mindfulness.

Step-by-Step Guide:

1. Perform simple movements like arm raises or head tilts.

2. Focus on your breath and the sensation of each movement.

3. Move slowly and deliberately.

4. Coordinate your breath with your movements.

5. Continue for 10-15 minutes.

8

---·---

ADVANCED EXERCISES

Embarking on advanced chair yoga exercises marks a significant milestone in one's yoga journey, especially for seniors who have embraced this practice as a part of their lifestyle. This 1000-word introduction will delve into the prerequisites and considerations necessary before transitioning to these advanced exercises, ensuring a safe and effective progression in one's yoga practice.

Before diving into advanced chair yoga, it's essential to have a solid foundation in basic and intermediate yoga exercises. This foundation includes not only familiarity with various yoga poses but also an understanding of one's body and its limitations. For seniors, this awareness is crucial as it helps prevent injuries and ensures that the exercises are performed effectively. Typically, someone ready for advanced chair yoga exercises would have consistently practiced chair yoga for an extended period, allowing their body to adapt and strengthen gradually.

The prerequisites for advanced chair yoga extend beyond physical readiness. They include a deepened sense of body awareness and the ability to maintain balance and coordination. Advanced exercises often involve more complex movements that require a good sense of balance to execute safely. Therefore, individuals should be comfortable with basic balance and strength exercises and possess the ability to hold poses for longer periods.

Flexibility plays a significant role in advancing one's yoga practice. Advanced chair yoga often incorporates poses that require a higher degree of flexibility, particularly in the spine, hips, and shoulders. While yoga, by nature, improves flexibility over time, those looking to advance their practice should already experience improved flexibility and a greater range of motion from their regular practice.

Another key prerequisite is an established mind-body connection. Advanced chair yoga is not just about performing more complex poses; it's about deepening the connection between the mind and the body. This connection allows practitioners to move with intention, understand the subtleties of each pose, and recognize the difference between a challenging stretch and discomfort that might lead to injury. A strong mind-body connection also enhances the ability to focus and remain present, which is essential in advanced practices where poses can be both physically and mentally challenging.

In addition to physical and mental readiness, individuals should also consider their overall health and any existing conditions. Seniors, in particular, might have health issues like osteoporosis, arthritis, or heart conditions that can affect their ability to perform certain yoga poses safely. It's crucial to consult with a healthcare provider before progressing to more advanced exercises, especially if there are any health concerns. Modifications and alternatives to certain poses can be made to accommodate individual health needs.

An often overlooked aspect before advancing in yoga is the understanding and practice of proper breathing techniques. Advanced chair yoga poses can be more physically demanding, and proper breathing is essential in executing these poses effectively and safely. Practitioners should be adept at using breath to guide their movements, maintain poses, and manage exertion.

It's also important to have the right mindset when approaching advanced chair yoga. This includes being patient with one's progress and understanding that advancing in yoga is not about achieving perfect poses but about the journey and what is learned along the way. It involves listening to the body, respecting its limits, and gradually pushing those limits to improve strength, flexibility, and balance.

Lastly, it's crucial to have the guidance of a qualified yoga instructor. Advanced chair yoga poses can be complex, and having an experienced instructor can provide the necessary guidance, adjustments, and insights to practice safely and effectively. An instructor can also offer personalized advice and modifications based on individual needs and abilities.

Advanced chair yoga offers a multitude of benefits, including enhanced physical strength, improved balance and flexibility, and deeper mental focus and relaxation. However, it's vital to approach this stage of yoga practice with caution, awareness, and respect for one's body and its capabilities. With the right preparation, mindset, and guidance, advancing in chair yoga can be a rewarding and enriching experience, leading to greater well-being and quality of life.

As practitioners embark on this advanced stage, they carry with them the lessons and strengths gained from their previous experiences. This journey into advanced chair yoga is not just a continuation of their physical practice, but a deeper exploration into the holistic benefits of yoga. It's a path that promises greater challenges but also greater rewards, as it opens up new possibilities for health, vitality, and inner peace.

1. Seated Eagle Pose

Step-by-Step Guide:

1. Sit upright, cross your right thigh over your left.

2. Hook your right foot behind your left calf, if possible.

3. Extend your arms straight, cross the left arm over the right, and bend your elbows.

4. Twist your arms so your palms meet.

5. Hold for several breaths, then switch sides.

2. Chair Warrior III

Step-by-Step Guide:

1. Stand behind the chair, holding onto the backrest.

2. Lean forward, lifting your left leg back, parallel to the floor.

3. Reach forward with your arms, keeping your body in a straight line.

4. Hold the pose, then switch legs.

3. Seated Half Moon Pose

Step-by-Step Guide:

1. Sit upright, extend your arms overhead.

2. Lean to the right, curving your spine into a crescent shape.

3. Hold the stretch, then lean to the left.

4. Seated Revolved Triangle

Step-by-Step Guide:

1. Sit sideways on the chair, legs extended.

2. Twist your torso to the right, reaching your left hand to your right foot.

3. Extend your right arm behind you, turning your head to look up.

4. Hold, then switch sides.

5. Chair Camel Pose

Step-by-Step Guide:

1. Kneel in front of the chair, feet hip-width apart.

2. Place your hands on the seat behind you.

3. Press your hips forward, arching your back and drop-

ping your head back.

4. Hold the pose for several breaths.

6. Seated Forward Bend with Leg Extension

Step-by-Step Guide:

1. Sit on the edge of the chair, extend your right leg.

2. Inhale and lengthen your spine.

3. Exhale and lean forward, reaching for your right foot.

4. Hold, then switch legs.

7. Chair Pigeon with Forward Bend

Step-by-Step Guide:

1. Sit, place your right ankle on your left knee.

2. Inhale and lengthen your spine.

3. Exhale and lean forward gently.

4. Hold, then switch sides.

8. Seated Spinal Twist with Leg Extension

Step-by-Step Guide:

> 1. Sit, extend your right leg.

> 2. Place your left foot outside your right thigh.

> 3. Twist to the left, using your right arm for leverage.

> 4. Hold, then switch sides.

9. Chair Warrior II

Step-by-Step Guide:

> 1. Sit sideways, extend your right leg out, left foot on the floor.

> 2. Open your arms wide, parallel to the floor.

> 3. Turn your head to look over your right hand.

> 4. Hold, then switch sides.

10. Seated Extended Side Angle

Step-by-Step Guide:

> 1. Sit sideways, extend your right leg, left knee bent.

> 2. Lean to the right, resting your right elbow on your thigh.

3. Extend your left arm overhead, creating a line from left foot to left hand.

4. Hold, then switch sides.

11. Chair Locust Pose

Step-by-Step Guide:

1. Sit at the edge of the chair, lean forward.

2. Extend your arms behind you, lifting them as you lean forward.

3. Lift your legs simultaneously, balancing on your abdomen.

4. Hold, then release.

12. Seated Boat Pose

Step-by-Step Guide:

1. Sit, hold onto the sides of the chair.

2. Lean back slightly, lift your feet off the floor.

3. Extend your legs and arms, balancing on your sit bones.

4. Hold, then release.

13. Chair Plank

Step-by-Step Guide:

    1. Stand facing the chair, place your hands on the seat.

    2. Step back until your body is in a straight line.

    3. Engage your core, keeping your body level.

    4. Hold, then release.

14. Seated Leg Lifts with Twist

Step-by-Step Guide:

    1. Sit upright, extend your right leg.

    2. Lift your leg, twisting your torso to the right.

    3. Return to center, then switch sides.

15. Chair Side Plank

Step-by-Step Guide:

    1. Sit sideways on the chair, legs together.

    2. Shift your weight to the right buttock, placing your right hand on the seat.

3. Lift your hips, extending your left arm up.

4. Hold, then switch sides.

16. Seated Cat-Cow with Leg Extension

Step-by-Step Guide:

1. Sit, extend your right leg.

2. Arch your back and look up (Cow).

3. Round your spine, tucking your chin (Cat).

4. Continue, alternating between Cow and Cat.

17. Chair Crescent Moon

Step-by-Step Guide:

1. Sit upright, extend your arms overhead.

2. Clasp your hands, lean to the right, creating a crescent shape.

3. Hold, then lean to the left.

18. Seated Warrior I

Step-by-Step Guide:

1. Sit facing forward, extend your right leg back.

2. Raise your arms overhead, palms facing each other.

3. Hold, then switch legs.

19. Chair Reverse Warrior

Step-by-Step Guide:

1. Sit sideways, extend your right leg, bend your left knee.

2. Place your left hand on the back of the chair, extend your right arm overhead.

3. Arch your back slightly, looking up.

4. Hold, then switch sides.

20. Seated Chair Bridge

Step-by-Step Guide:

1. Sit, feet flat, hands on the seat behind you.

2. Press into your hands and feet, lifting your hips.

3. Keep your neck relaxed, shoulders away from ears.

4. Hold, then lower back down.

21. Seated Half Lord of the Fishes

Step-by-Step Guide:

1. Sit upright, legs extended.

2. Bend your right knee, placing your foot flat on the floor outside your left thigh.

3. Twist to the right, placing your left elbow outside your right knee.

4. Hold the twist, then switch sides.

22. Chair Sun Salutations

Step-by-Step Guide:

1. Sit upright, inhale and raise your arms overhead.

2. Exhale, fold forward, reaching towards your toes.

3. Inhale, rise halfway, lengthening your spine.

4. Exhale, fold forward again.

5. Inhale, rise to a seated position, arms overhead.

6. Exhale, lower arms to your sides.

23. Seated Tree Pose

Step-by-Step Guide:

   1. Sit upright, place your right foot on your left thigh.

   2. Press your foot and thigh together, finding balance.

   3. Raise your arms overhead, palms together.

   4. Hold the pose, then switch legs.

24. Chair Downward Dog

Step-by-Step Guide:

   1. Stand facing the chair, hands on the seat.

   2. Walk your feet back, folding at the hips.

   3. Press your hands into the chair, extending your spine.

   4. Hold the pose, feeling the stretch in your back.

25. Seated Side Plank

Step-by-Step Guide:

   1. Sit sideways, legs together, weight on your right buttock.

   2. Place your right hand on the seat, lift your hips.

3. Extend your left arm up, body in a straight line.

4. Hold, then switch sides.

26. Chair Triangle Pose

Step-by-Step Guide:

1. Sit sideways, right leg extended, left foot flat.

2. Extend your right arm towards your right foot.

3. Raise your left arm, opening your chest.

4. Hold, then switch sides.

27. Seated Forward Bend with Twist

Step-by-Step Guide:

1. Sit upright, legs extended.

2. Inhale, lengthen your spine.

3. Exhale, fold forward and twist to the right.

4. Hold, then twist to the left on the next fold.

28. Chair Cow Face Arms

Step-by-Step Guide:

1. Sit upright, extend your right arm up, bend at the elbow.

2. Bring your left arm behind your back, bend at the elbow.

3. Clasp your hands if possible, stretching your arms.

4. Hold, then switch arms.

29. Seated Warrior Flow

Step-by-Step Guide:

1. Sit sideways, right leg extended, left knee bent.

2. Flow between Warrior II and Reverse Warrior poses.

3. Hold each pose for a few breaths, then switch sides.

30. Chair Upward Plank

Step-by-Step Guide:

1. Sit, hands on the seat behind you, fingers pointing forward.

2. Press into your hands and feet, lifting your hips.

3. Keep your legs and arms straight, head relaxed.

4. Hold, then lower back down.

31. Seated Leg Lift and Twist

Step-by-Step Guide:

1. Sit upright, extend your right leg.

2. Lift the leg, twist your torso to the right.

3. Return to center, then switch legs.

32. Chair Lunge Twist

Step-by-Step Guide:

1. Stand facing the chair, step back with your right foot.

2. Bend your left knee, enter a lunge position.

3. Twist your torso to the left, extending your arms.

4. Hold, then switch sides.

33. Seated Eagle Arms with Forward Bend

Step-by-Step Guide:

1. Sit upright, cross your right arm over your left at the elbows.

2. Twist your arms so your palms meet.

3. Inhale, then exhale and fold forward.

4. Hold, then rise and switch arms.

34. Chair Supported Bridge Pose

Step-by-Step Guide:

1. Sit, then turn and lie back on the chair.

2. Rest your upper back on the chair, feet flat on the floor.

3. Press into your feet, lifting your hips.

4. Hold, then slowly lower down.

35. Seated Side Leg Raise

Step-by-Step Guide:

1. Sit sideways, right leg on the chair, left leg hanging off.

2. Slowly raise your left leg to the side.

3. Hold, then lower and switch legs.

9

---·---

ADDITIONAL RESOURCES

These resources offer a mix of practical guidance, philosophical insights, and community support, catering to the diverse needs and interests of senior chair yoga practitioners.

1. **"Chair Yoga: Seated Exercises for Health and Wellbeing" by Edeltraud Rohnfeld**: A book offering a comprehensive guide to chair yoga, ideal for beginners and seniors.

2. **Yoga Journal**: An online and print magazine providing a wealth of information on yoga, including articles, videos, and tips for practitioners at all levels.

3. **"Relax into Yoga for Seniors: A Six-Week Program for Strength, Balance, Flexibility, and Pain Relief" by Kimberly Carson and Carol Krucoff**: This book offers a tailored yoga program for seniors focusing on strength, balance, and flexibility.

4. **Yoga With Adriene (YouTube Channel)**: Popular online yoga instructor Adriene Mishler offers a variety of yoga videos, including some suitable for seniors or those with limited mobility.

5. **SilverSneakers**: A fitness program for seniors that offers yoga classes among other health and fitness resources.

6. **"The New Yoga for Healthy Aging" by Suza Francina**: A book focusing on yoga practices that promote healthy aging and vitality.

7. **Mindful Yoga Academy**: Offers online resources and classes focusing on mindful yoga, suitable for seniors and those seeking a gentle approach.

8. **Yoga Alliance**: A large yoga organization that provides resources and directories for yoga classes and instructors, useful for finding senior-friendly classes.

9. **"Anatomy of Movement" by Blandine Calais-Germain**: This book offers insights into how the body moves, which can be helpful in understanding and improving yoga practice.

10. **Senior Yoga Community Groups (Facebook and Meetup)**: Online platforms where seniors practicing yoga can connect, share experiences, and find support.

11. **"Yoga for Seniors with Jane Adams"**: A series of DVDs offering yoga routines designed specifically for seniors.

12. **Gaia**: An online platform offering yoga and meditation videos, including sessions suitable for older adults.

13. **"Chair Yoga for You: A Practical Guide" by Betsy Trapasso**: A guidebook that offers various chair yoga routines and the benefits associated with them.

14. **Daily Yoga App**: A mobile app offering a variety of yoga classes and routines, with options for all levels.

15. **"Yoga Over 50" by Mary Stewart**: This book provides modified yoga practices for older practitioners.

16. **Yoga International**: An online resource offering articles, classes, and workshops on yoga, meditation, and holistic health.

17. **"Yoga and the Wisdom of Menopause" by Suza Francina**: A book exploring how yoga can support women through menopause, including chair yoga options.

18. **Headspace (Meditation App)**: While primarily a meditation app, Headspace also offers mindful movement and yoga sessions.

19. **"The Gentle Way of Hatha Yoga" by Laurie Sanford**: This book emphasizes gentle yoga practices, suitable for seniors and beginners.

20. **Insight Timer (Meditation App)**: Offers guided meditations and talks, some of which are focused on movement and yoga.

21. **"Chair Vinyasa: Yoga Flow for Every Body" by Olivia Miller**: A guide to creating fluid yoga sequences using a chair.

22. **National Center for Complementary and Integrative Health**: Provides research-based information on yoga's health benefits.

23. **"The Heart of Yoga: Developing a Personal Practice" by T.K.V. Desikachar**: Offers insights into personalizing yoga practice, relevant for seniors adapting yoga to their needs.

24. **Yoga for Seniors Certification Programs**: Programs for yoga instructors focusing on teaching yoga to seniors, useful for those looking to specialize.

25. **"Teaching Yoga: Essential Foundations and Techniques" by Mark Stephens**: A comprehensive guide on teaching yoga, with relevant information for those instructing seniors.

26. **YogaDownload.com**: An online platform with a variety of yoga classes, including chair yoga options.

27. **"Accessible Yoga: Poses and Practices for Every Body" by Jivana Heyman**: Focuses on making yoga inclusive, with sections on chair yoga.

28. **DoYogaWithMe (Online Yoga Platform)**: Offers a wide range of yoga videos, including classes suitable for older adults.

29. **"Light on Yoga" by B.K.S. Iyengar**: A classic yoga text that, while not specific to chair yoga, provides a deep understanding of yoga philosophy and practice.

30. **YogaGlo**: An online yoga platform with a diverse range of classes, including ones focused on gentle and senior yoga.

Made in the USA
Coppell, TX
24 June 2024